HARD FACTS IN
ORTHOPAEDICS

HARD FACTS IN
ORTHOPAEDICS

Robert C. Schenck, Jr., M.D.

Assistant Professor, Department of Orthopaedics,
The University of Texas Health Science Center at San Antonio,
San Antonio, Texas

ILLUSTRATED BY

William M. Winn

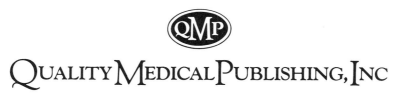

QUALITY MEDICAL PUBLISHING, INC

ST. LOUIS, MISSOURI
1993

Printed in the United States of America

PUBLISHER Karen Berger

PROJECT MANAGER Carolita Deter

MANUSCRIPT EDITOR Rose Mary Goerke

PRODUCTION Kay Ehsani, Susan Trail, Judy Bamert

BOOK DESIGN Susan Trail

COVER DESIGN Diane M. Beasley

Quality Medical Publishing, Inc.
11970 Borman Drive, Suite 222
St. Louis, Missouri 63146

LIBRARY OF CONGRESS CATALOGING-IN-PUBLICATION DATA
Schenck, Robert C.
    Hard facts in orthopaedics / Robert C. Schenck, Jr. ; illustrated
by William M. Winn.
        p.   cm.
    Includes bibliographical references and index.
    ISBN 0-942219-46-5
    1. Orthopedics—Handbooks, manuals, etc. 2. Musculoskeletal
system—Anatomy—Handbooks, manuals, etc. 3. Fractures—
Classification—Handbooks, manuals, etc. 4. Bones—Metabolism—
Disorders—Handbooks, manuals, etc. I. Title.
    [DNLM: 1. Bone Diseases, Metabolic. 2. Fractures—classification.
3. Musculoskeletal System—anatomy & histology. WE 168 S324h 1993]
RD732.5.S34   1993
617.3—dc20
DNLM/DLC
for Library of Congress   92-48563
                                   CIP

QM/M/M
5   4   3   2   1

TO MY FAMILY

my wife
for her love and friendship

my parents
for their support and guidance

my children
for making it all worthwhile

PREFACE

This book is derived from a series of notes and observations that I developed throughout my residency in an attempt to summarize the essentials of orthopaedics. My goal was to convert the notes into a text that would be suitable for both the desk and the pocket. The first section describes and classifies some of the basic components of the discipline with special reference to the musculoskeletal and fracture anatomies. The text also includes an explanation of metabolic bone disease that I have found extremely useful in the teaching and understanding of this complicated process.

The book is designed to serve as a concise and accessible reference for students of orthopaedics, both young and old.

Robert C. Schenck, Jr.

ACKNOWLEDGMENTS

I am indebted to many individuals for the successful completion of this text. I would like to thank my wife for her constant support and dependable advice. Support by Teri Hill, even after numerous revisions, was without a doubt another key to the success of the project. I am greatly indebted to James D. Heckman, M.D., Chairman of the Department of Orthopaedic Surgery at the University of Texas Health Science Center at San Antonio, who gave initial direction. Furthermore, my publisher, Karen Berger, with her infectious energy and undying support, made preparation of the book a pleasure. Bill Winn also played a critical role by creating the superb illustrations. In addition, I would like to thank Joseph Moskal, M.D., for my early education in metabolic bone disease. Finally, I would like to acknowledge the many dedicated teachers who were instrumental in my education, instilling in me the desire to teach.

CONTENTS

HARD FACTS IN
ORTHOPAEDICS

1

ANATOMY

UPPER EXTREMITY
Brachial Plexus

This intricate structure surrounding the axillary artery is an ideal source for examination questions. A gentle warning should preface this discussion—know the brachial plexus anatomy thoroughly and be prepared to draw the structure from memory for written examinations. Drawing the structure from memory is very helpful for recall purposes also. When given a test booklet, draw out the plexus; in effect, this gives you a reference when moderately exhausted after hours of test taking.

The brachial plexus is described in five stages outlined below and in Fig. 1. The stages are *roots*, *trunks*, *divisions*, *cords*, and peripheral nerves. If the word "branches" is substituted for "peripheral nerves," the mnemonic "Robert Taylor drinks cold beer" can be useful.

The five stages are as follows:
1. Undivided ventral *rami* or roots
2. Formation of three *trunks* (superior, middle, inferior)
3. *Division* of each trunk into anterior and posterior aspects
4. Union of divisions into *cords* (medial, posterior, lateral)
5. Derivation of principal *nerves* from the cords

After passing between the scalene muscles, the rami form trunks; each trunk is derived from a specific cervical level(s):

Superior	C5 to C6
Middle	C7
Inferior	C8 to T1

The third stage (division) designates nerves supplying ventral and dorsal motor units. The anterior and posterior divisions of the brachial plexus from C5 to C7 are approximately equal in size. The posterior division of the inferior trunk (C8) is small. The fourth stage (cords) is subdivided into the medial, posterior, and lateral aspects based on position to the axillary artery. (NOTE: Cords are at the level of the axillary artery that is crossed by the pectoralis minor musculature and designated the "second part"; the "first part" of the axillary artery extends from the first rib to the upper edge of the pectoralis minor; the "third part" extends from the axillary border of pectoralis minor to the inferior border of teres major.)

Lateral cord	C5 to C7
Posterior cord	C5 to T1
Medial cord	C8 to T1

Before discussing specific branches of the plexus, a brief description of the subclavian arterial anatomy is necessary. The right subclavian artery is a branch of the brachiocephalic artery; the left is an independent branch of the aortic arch. The subclavian artery crosses between the anterior and middle scalene muscles at the level of the clavicle.

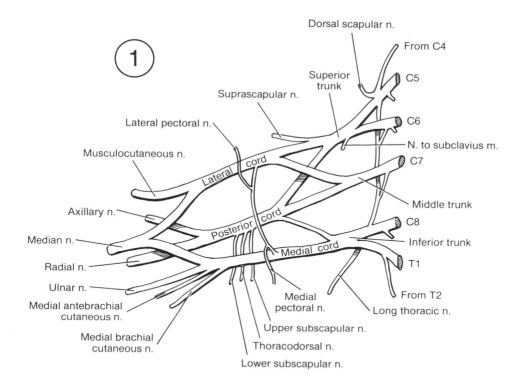

Muscular branches

Muscular branches to the anterior, middle, and posterior scalene muscles originate from the lower four cervical nerves as they exit the intervertebral foramen. A branch of C5 contributes to the phrenic nerve at the lateral border of the anterior scalene muscle. Other branches arising from the proximal portion of the brachial plexus are grouped topographically according to their position to the clavicle—supraclavicular or infraclavicular.

The nerves arising from the *supraclavicular branches* are as follows:

Dorsal scapular nerve (C5): Supplies the rhomboid and levator scapular muscles after passing through the middle scalene muscle.

Long thoracic nerve (C5 to C7): Innervates the serratus anterior muscle; the neurovascular bundle comprises the long thoracic nerve and the lateral thoracic artery. Branches of this nerve from C5 and C6 pass through the scalenus medius (middle) muscle, whereas the branch of C7 passes over the first rib.

Nerve to subclavius

Suprascapular nerve (C5-6): Supplies the supraspinatus and infraspinatus muscles. The nerve passes anterior to the trapezius; after innervating the supraspinatus, it travels into the suprascapular notch under the transverse scapular ligament. The suprascapular artery passes over the transverse scapular ligament.

The nerves arising from the *infraclavicular branches* are as follows:

Lateral pectoral nerve: Arises from the lateral cord (specifically, C5 to C7) and forms a loop with the medial pectoral nerve.

Medial pectoral nerve: Arises from medial cord (C8 and T1)—Pectoralis major, lateral and medial pectoral nerve; pectoralis minor, medial pectoral nerve.

Medial brachial cutaneous nerve: Arises from medial cord (C8 and T1) and is responsible for sensation of the posterior aspect of the lower portion of the arm to the olecranon.

Medial antebrachial cutaneous nerve: Also arises from the medial cord (C8 and T1) and provides sensation for the medial volar forearm.

Subscapular nerve: Arises from the posterior cord and is made up of the following three branches—

1. Upper subscapular nerve (C5-6) innervates subscapularis
2. Middle subscapular nerve (C7-8) (a.k.a. thoracodorsal nerve) innervates the latissimus dorsi
3. Lower subscapular nerve (C5-6) innervates the teres major and subscapularis

NOTE: Subscapularis is innervated by the upper and lower subscapular nerves.

Axillary nerve: A branch of the posterior cord, the axillary nerve travels through the quadrangular space with the posterior circumflex humeral artery.

Fig. 2 further illustrates the anatomy of the brachial plexus. The ability to draw the entire structure from memory is essential.

Hand

The palm is divided into three compartments: hypothenar, central, and thenar. The central compartment contains the eight finger flexors and the flexor pollicis longus muscle. The central compartment is separated into two potential spaces—dorsal to the flexors and palmar to the interossei muscles—namely, the midpalmar and thenar spaces. The midpalmar space drains the ring and long finger flexor sheaths, whereas the thenar space drains the index finger and thumb.

The thenar and hypothenar compartments are located on the palmar side of the hand. Each group contains an abductor, opponens, and flexor. The origins include the flexor retinaculum and transverse carpal ligament; thenar muscles originate from the scaphoid and trapezium, and the hypothenar muscles originate from the hamate and pisiform bones.

Insertions are similar and easily remembered. The flexor and abductor insert on the base of the proximal phalanx. The opponens pollicis inserts along the metacarpal shaft. Function of the opponens brings the thumb into the palm of the hand through thumb abduction, flexion, and pronation.

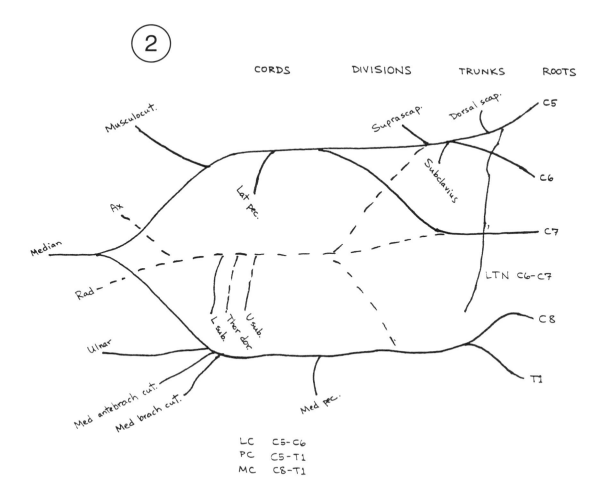

(2)

CORDS   DIVISIONS   TRUNKS   ROOTS

LC   C5–C6
PC   C5–T1
MC   C8–T1

Interossei muscles

Dorsally, there are four muscles (bipennate) that originate from both metacarpals (remember "DAB" for *d*orsal *ab*ductors).

Palmarly, there are three muscles (unipennate) that originate from one metacarpal (remember "PAD" for *p*almar *ad*ductors). Study Figs. 3 and 4.

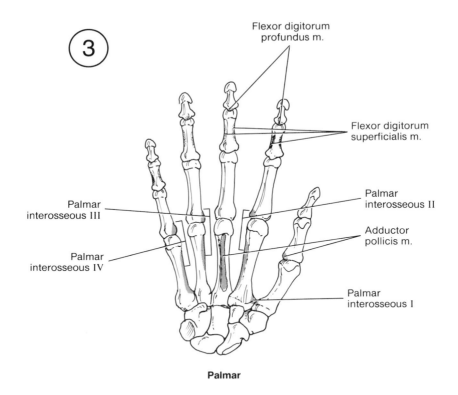

Palmar

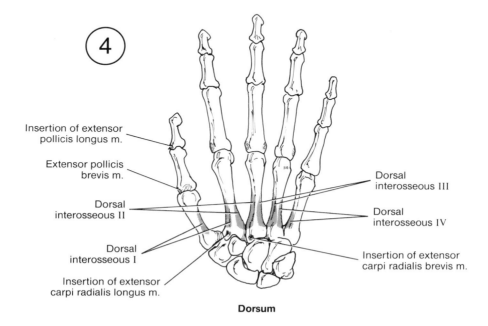

Dorsum

Arterial supply

The arterial supply of the thumb is from the deep palmar arch. The remaining four digits receive their arterial supply from the superficial arch. The deep arch is proximal to the superficial arch (and obviously deep or dorsal). The deep arch lies dorsal to the long flexors under cover of the palmar interosseous fascia. The deep arch gives off the princeps pollicis, indicis proprius, and metacarpal branches. The metacarpal branches join the more palmar common digital arteries to pass between the natatory ligament and deep metacarpal ligament on into the fingers. The superficial palmar arch is formed by the ulnar and superficial radial arteries (Fig. 5).

Questions concerning the median nerve anatomy of the hand are usually straightforward despite the complex variations of the recurrent motor branch. The most common takeoff of the motor branch from the median nerve is palmar or radiopalmar.

The radial nerve does not innervate the intrinsic muscles of the hand.

The ulnar nerve has a complex anatomy that will be reviewed in detail. In the proximal forearm the ulnar nerve passes between the two heads of the flexor carpi ulnaris; it then travels under the cover of the flexor carpi ulnaris lying on the flexor digitorum profundus. At the wrist the anatomic alignment from the ulnar to the radial position is (1) flexor carpi ulnaris, (2) ulnar nerve, and (3) ulnar artery. The forearm is "framed" by nerves—that is, the ulnar and radial nerves are ulnar and radial, respectively, to their accompanying artery. Two inches proximal to the wrist, the dorsal cutaneous branch (supplying the dorsal aspect of the ring and little fingers proximal to the midpoint of the

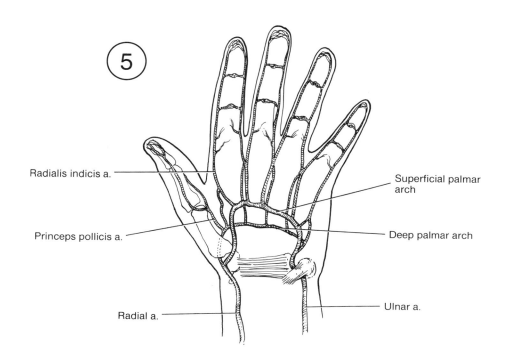

Radialis indicis a.

Princeps pollicis a.

Radial a.

Superficial palmar arch

Deep palmar arch

Ulnar a.

middle phalanges) of the ulnar nerve splits off the parent trunk. Along the radial aspect of the pisiform, the ulnar nerve divides into its superficial and deep branches.

The superficial branch innervates the palmaris brevis and then supplies cutaneous sensation to the ring and little fingers. The deep branch sinks into the palm between the flexor digiti minimi and abductor digiti minimi. It perforates the opponens digiti minimi and follows the deep palmar arch. The deep branch supplies the following muscles: the abductor digiti minimi, flexor digiti minimi brevis, opponens digiti minimi, all interossei, ulnar two lumbricales, adductor pollicis, and deep head of the flexor pollicis brevis (conceptually the first interosseus).

Surgical Exposures

Surgical approaches of the shoulder, humerus, elbow, forearm, and wrist should be conceptualized as a whole. This is especially helpful for the area around the elbow.

Shoulder and proximal humerus

The anterior approach proximally is through the deltopectoral groove. More distal exposure of the humerus is gained by splitting the brachialis (medial head, musculocutaneous innervation; lateral head, radial nerve).

Study the three diagrams provided in Figs. 6 through 8.

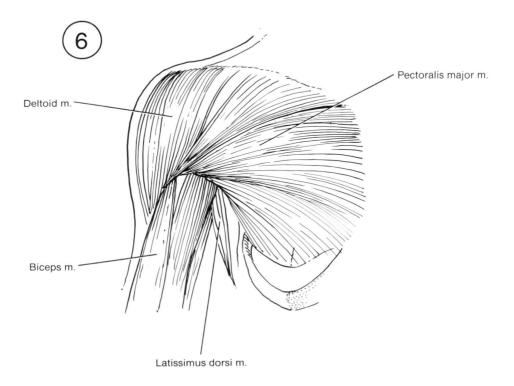

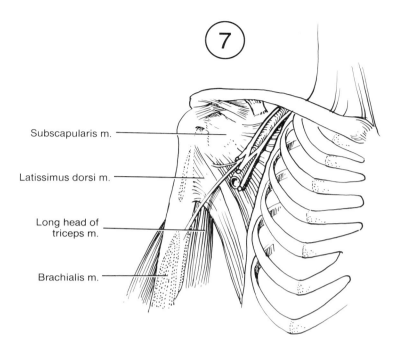

Subscapularis m.

Latissimus dorsi m.

Long head of
triceps m.

Brachialis m.

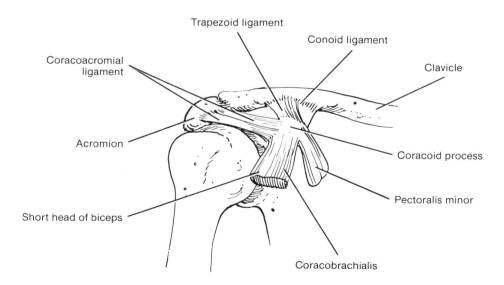

Trapezoid ligament

Conoid ligament

Coracoacromial
ligament

Clavicle

Acromion

Coracoid process

Short head of biceps

Pectoralis minor

Coracobrachialis

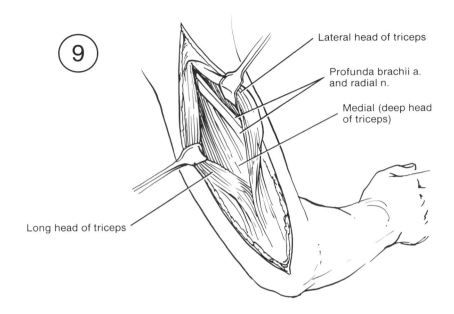

Lateral head of triceps

Profunda brachii a. and radial n.

Medial (deep head of triceps)

Long head of triceps

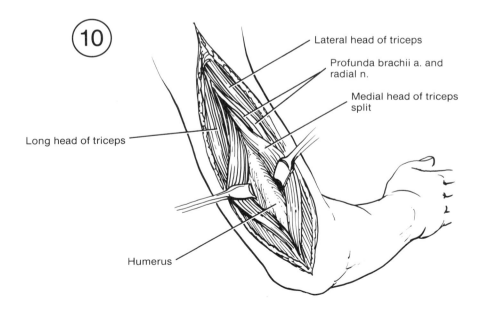

Lateral head of triceps

Profunda brachii a. and radial n.

Medial head of triceps split

Long head of triceps

Humerus

The posterior approach to the humerus, the triceps splitting approach (Figs. 9 and 10), allows access to its lower three fourths. There are two layers to the approach: superficial and deep. Superficially, the long (origin: infraglenoid tubercle of scapula) and lateral (origin: lateral lip of spiral groove) heads of the triceps are split. The inner layer is the medial head of the triceps (inferomedial to the spiral groove), which is split to expose the humerus. The radial nerve and profunda brachii artery separate the lateral and medial heads.

It is helpful to split the long and lateral heads proximally (superficial layer), working distally into the common insertion. When splitting the medial head of the triceps, it is important to remain subperiosteal. Straying medially into the medial head of the triceps can injure the ulnar nerve as it pierces the medial intramuscular septum. The posterior approach to the elbow is the transolecranon (osteotomy) approach or the triceps subperiosteal exposure described by Bryan and Morrey.

Distal humerus (Figs. 11 through 13)

The anterolateral approach to the distal humerus is as follows. The internervous plane is between the brachialis and brachioradialis. Superficially, look for the *lateral* antebrachial cutaneous nerve as it crosses the surgical field (this nerve exits between the brachialis and biceps). Next, identify the radial nerve under the cover of the brachioradialis. Distal exposure (into the elbow) is through its anterolateral internervous plane, that of the brachioradialis and pronator teres. With the anterolateral approach to the capitellum, ligation of the radial recurrent artery is often needed. Detachment of the supinator muscle (in forearm supination) is required for exposure of the proximal radius (Fig. 13).

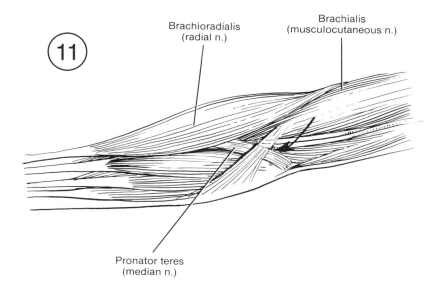

Brachioradialis
(radial n.)

Brachialis
(musculocutaneous n.)

11

Pronator teres
(median n.)

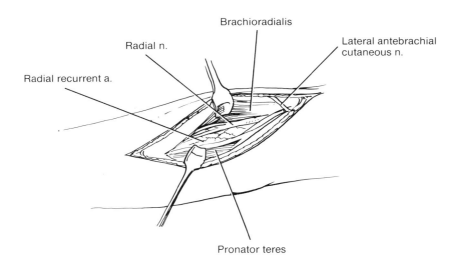

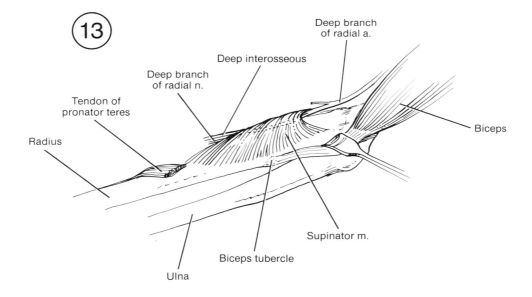

Elbow

Before moving to the forearm, the elbow approaches can be studied by a discussion of the anterior, medial, and posterolateral approaches.

The anterior approach to the elbow fossa requires incision of the lacertus fibrosus and follows the neurovascular bundle medially between the pronator teres and the brachialis. Proximal exposure of the distal humerus (medial) through this approach travels between the triceps and the brachialis. The medial approach to the elbow uses the pronator teres/brachialis interval with osteotomy of the flexor pronator group. Study Figs. 14 and 15.

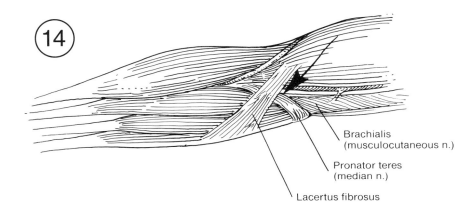

Brachialis
(musculocutaneous n.)

Pronator teres
(median n.)

Lacertus fibrosus

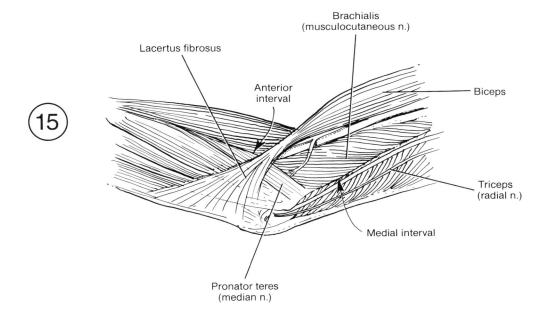

Brachialis
(musculocutaneous n.)

Lacertus fibrosus

Anterior
interval

Biceps

Triceps
(radial n.)

Medial interval

Pronator teres
(median n.)

The lateral approach to the distal humerus is between the internervous plane of the triceps and brachioradialis (Kocher approach). This cannot be extended proximally because the radial nerve pierces the lateral intermuscular septum and is at risk for injury. See Figs. 16 and 17.

Distal extension of the lateral approach into the elbow joint is through the posterolateral approach to the elbow. This uses the plane between the anconeus and the extensor carpi ulnaris. Forearm pronation is performed to move the posterior interosseous nerve away from the surgical field. Note Fig. 18. Thus the Kocher approach is extended distally through the posterolateral plane. This distal exposure cannot be taken past the annular ligament for risk of injury to the posterior interosseous nerve.

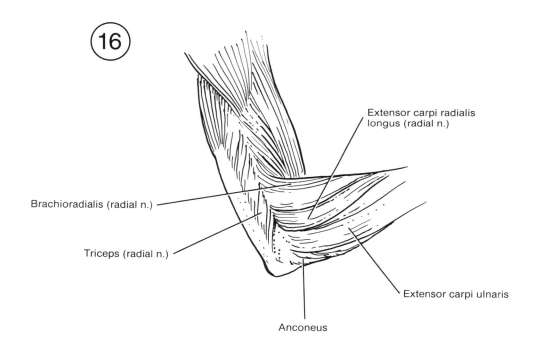

(16)

Extensor carpi radialis longus (radial n.)

Brachioradialis (radial n.)

Triceps (radial n.)

Extensor carpi ulnaris

Anconeus

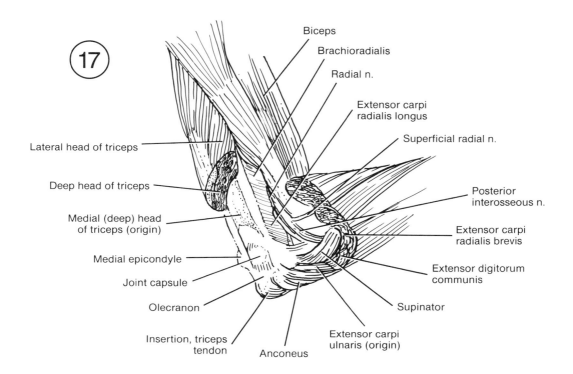

(17)

Biceps

Brachioradialis

Radial n.

Extensor carpi
radialis longus

Superficial radial n.

Lateral head of triceps

Deep head of triceps

Medial (deep) head
of triceps (origin)

Medial epicondyle

Joint capsule

Olecranon

Insertion, triceps
tendon

Anconeus

Extensor carpi
ulnaris (origin)

Supinator

Extensor digitorum
communis

Extensor carpi
radialis brevis

Posterior
interosseous n.

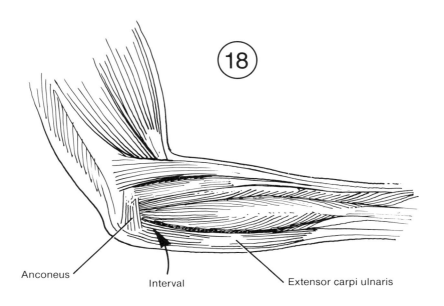

(18)

Anconeus

Interval

Extensor carpi ulnaris

Forearm

Moving into the forearm, the radius is most easily exposed by the anterior approach of Henry. This approach uses the muscle interval of the brachioradialis (radially) and the pronator teres and flexor carpi radialis (ulnarly). Deep dissection requires sharp detachment of the supinator (with the forearm supinated) and the pronator teres (with the forearm pronated) followed by the flexor digitorum superficialis, flexor pollicis longus, and, most distally, the pronator quadratus. Note Figs. 19 and 20.

The dorsal approach (Fig. 21) to the radius (Thompson) travels between the extensor carpi radialis brevis (radially) and the extensor digitorum communis and extensor pollicis longus muscles ulnarly. The posterior interosseus nerve must be identified (by dissecting it out of the supinator) before the supinator muscle can be detached.

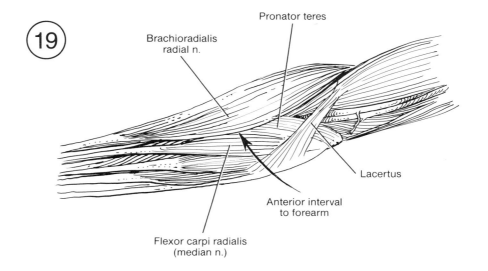

19

Brachioradialis
radial n.

Pronator teres

Lacertus

Anterior interval
to forearm

Flexor carpi radialis
(median n.)

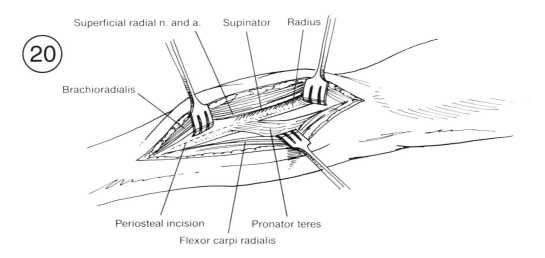

20

Superficial radial n. and a.   Supinator   Radius

Brachioradialis

Periosteal incision   Pronator teres

Flexor carpi radialis

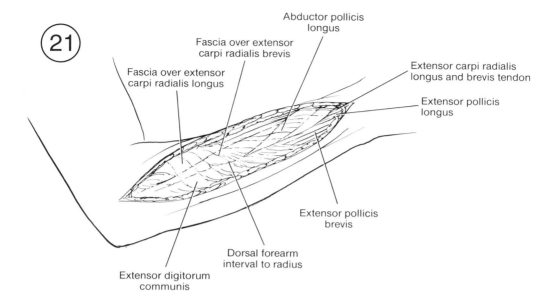

Abductor pollicis
longus

Fascia over extensor
carpi radialis brevis

Fascia over extensor
carpi radialis longus

Extensor carpi radialis
longus and brevis tendon

Extensor pollicis
longus

Extensor pollicis
brevis

Dorsal forearm
interval to radius

Extensor digitorum
communis

Wrist

The volar approach (Fig. 22) to the scaphoid is the distal most extension of the anterior forearm exposure and is between the flexor carpi radialis muscle and radial artery.

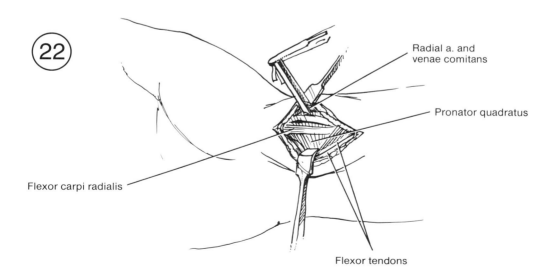

Radial a. and
venae comitans

Pronator quadratus

Flexor carpi radialis

Flexor tendons

Lastly, the dorsal approach to the scaphoid is over the snuff box between the tendons of the extensor pollicis longus and extensor pollicis brevis superficially. The extensor pollicis longus and the extensor carpi radialis longus are mobilized, and the tendons are retracted ulnarly; the radial artery and extensor pollicis brevis are retracted together radially. NOTE: The dorsal approach to the scaphoid can endanger the dorsal carpal branch of the radial artery, which supplies the proximal two thirds of the scaphoid (Figs. 23 and 24).

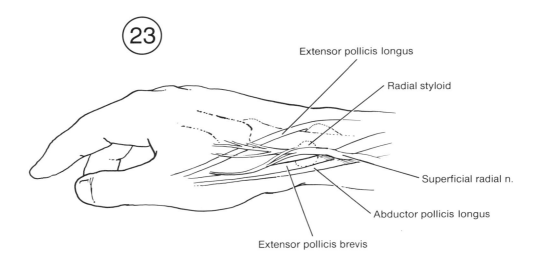

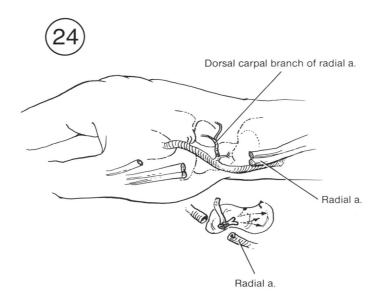

SPINE
Nerve Root

You must know the anatomy of the nerve root complex, specifically with respect to the level at which the nerve root exits, and you should be able to predict which motor function (therefore nerve root) is affected based on a radiographic study documenting a herniated disk. Thus it is necessary to know the segmental innervation of the upper and lower extremity musculature and the corresponding level of exit of the nerve root from the intervertebral foramen.

The easiest way to remember corresponding levels is not through a numeric system but rather to remember two specific facts: (1) the first cervical nerve root exits from under the skull and (2) there are eight cervical roots. With these facts in mind, you can work down the spine and place each nerve at its corresponding motion segment. Which nerve root exits at the C3-4 intervertebral foramen? Working down from the skull (when C1 exits), you will realize that the nerve root at the C3-4 interspace is C4. The C7-T1 interspace is the location of the eighth cervical nerve. From the thoracic spine caudally, the nerve root level corresponds to the upper vertebral body of the interspace. The third thoracic root exits at the 3-4 thoracic level. This carries into the lumbar area where, for instance, the fourth lumbar nerve exits at the L4-5 interspace. Disk pathology at the lumbar level can be correlated to root involvement by the anatomic fact that each root exits under the pedicle of the upper body (Fig. 25). Thus a herniated disk at L4-5 will "pinch" the fifth lumbar root; the fourth lumbar root has exited under the L4 pedicle *above* the ruptured L4-5 disk. Nerve involvement in spondylolisthesis usually affects the root at that level: L4-5 listhesis affects L4; L5-S1 listhesis affects L5.

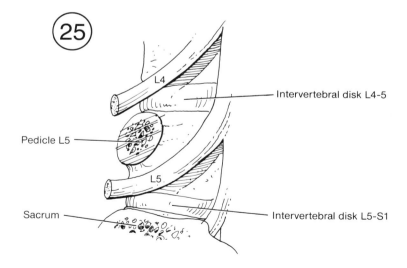

Surgical Exposures
Cervical spine

The posterior approach to the cervical spine can be used for any level. When exposing the posterior arches of the atlas and axis, careful stripping of the lateral aspects is required to prevent injury to the vertebral artery. In addition, care must be taken to protect the occipital nerves supplying sensation to the posterior aspect of the skull (Fig. 26).

The anterior approach to the cervical spine from C3 to T1 will be outlined. This approach can be used to gain access to the odontoid, but it is a complicated procedure.

The landmarks of cervical levels are as follows:

Lower border of mandible   C2-3
Thyroid cartilage   C4-5
Cricoid cartilage   C6

Either side of the neck can be used; however, the left side is recommended because of potential damage to the right recurrent laryngeal nerve. The left recurrent laryngeal nerve ascends between the esophagus and trachea after branching from the vagus

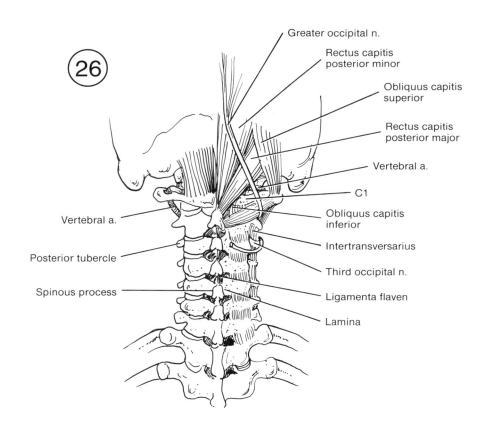

nerve at the aorta. On the right side the recurrent laryngeal nerve runs alongside the trachea after hooking over the subclavian artery. In the lower aspect of the right-sided approach, the recurrent laryngeal nerve runs from the lateral to medial aspect and is at risk for injury. Thus use of the left side is recommended in this approach.

Make a transverse incision on the skin at the level of pathology (see landmarks listed on p. 20), followed by incising the platysma muscle longitudinally along its fibers. The plane of dissection is between the sternocleidomastoid and longus colli. Incise the anterior border of the sternocleidomastoid fascia and retract this muscle and the carotid sheath laterally. Retract the strap muscles, trachea, and esophagus medially. Carefully incise the pretrachial fascia to separate the carotid sheath from the trachea and esophagus. The superior and inferior thyroid arteries can limit proximal exposure and are divided if needed. Incise the longus colli in the midline to expose the vertebral body and disk space. Note that the longus colli muscles lie on each side of the vertebral body with overlying sympathetic chains. (Injury to the sympathetic nerves results in Horner's syndrome; use the mnemonic "HAMP" for *H*orner's: *a*nhydrosis, *m*yosis, *p*tosis.) Place retractors under the longus colli when retracting structures medially to prevent injury to the recurrent laryngeal nerve. Last, the vertebral artery is lateral to the exposure (and anterior to the nerve roots) (Figs. 27 and 28).

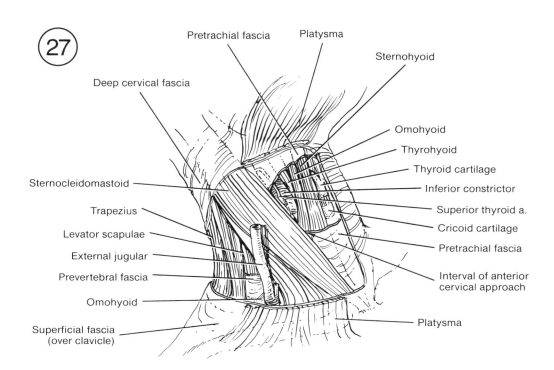

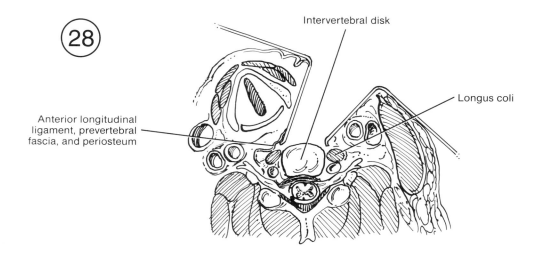

Thoracic spine

The costotransversectomy approach to the vertebral body requires removal of a portion of the rib and transverse process. Reflecting the pleura allows exposure of the lateral edge of the vertebral body (Fig. 29).

Lumbar spine

Approach to the L5-S1 interspace (for incision and drainage) is usually made transperitoneally. For other lumbar levels, however, the retroperitoneal (or anterolateral) approach is used (Fig. 30). The patient is in the lateral decubitus position with the left side up (aorta is closer and more resistant to tearing than the vena cava). Once the skin incision is made, incise the three muscle layers of the external oblique, internal oblique, and transversalis fascia. Retract the peritoneum anteriorly. The ureter retracts with these contents since it is loosely attached to the peritoneum. The genitofemoral nerve (cremaster muscle and groin sensation) lies on the anteromedial surface of the psoas and is attached to the fascia. Also note that the sympathetic chain lies on the lateral aspect of the vertebral body (and most medial on the psoas).

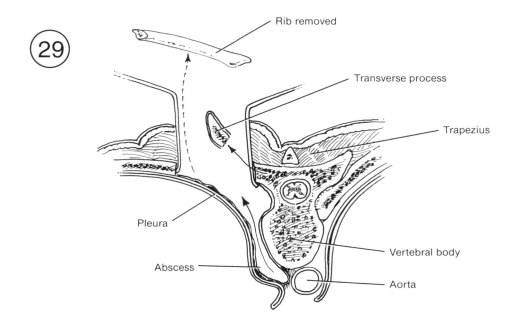

29

Rib removed

Transverse process

Trapezius

Pleura

Abscess

Vertebral body

Aorta

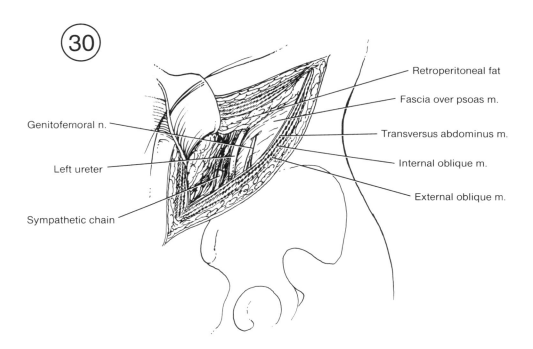

30

Retroperitoneal fat

Fascia over psoas m.

Genitofemoral n.

Transversus abdominus m.

Left ureter

Internal oblique m.

External oblique m.

Sympathetic chain

PELVIS AND LOWER EXTREMITY
Lumbosacral Plexus (Fig. 31)

The lumbar plexus includes the ventral roots from L1 to L4. Motor innervation is as follows: psoas major, L2 to L4; psoas minor, L1 to L2; iliacus, femoral nerve L2 to L4. The ventral rami of L2 to L4 have anterior and posterior divisions forming two nerves: the obturator nerve L2 to L4 (anterior) and femoral nerve L2 to L4 (posterior).

The sacral plexus includes the roots from L4 to S4. Nerves formed by this plexus include:

Sciatic
   Preaxial: Tibial portion L4 to S1
   Postaxial: Common peroneal portion L4 to S1
Superior gluteal nerve: L4 to S1
Inferior gluteal nerve: L5 to S2

The nerve root common to both the lumbar plexus and sacral plexus is L4.

Lumbar Plexus	
Iliohypogastric nerve	L1 (T12)
Ilioinguinal nerve	L1
Genitofemoral nerve	L1, 2
Lateral femoral cutaneous nerve	L2, 3
Obturator nerve	L2, 3, 4
Accessory obturator nerve	L3, 4
Femoral nerve	L2, 3, 4
Sacral Plexus	
Sciatic nerve	L4, 5, S1, 2, 3
Muscular branches	
To piriformis	S1, 2
To levator ani and coccygeus	S3, 4
Superior gluteal nerve	L4, 5, S1
Inferior gluteal nerve	L5, S1, 2
Nerve to obturator femoris and inferior gemellus muscles	L4, 5, S1
Nerve to obturator internus and superior gemellus muscles	L5, S1, 2
Posterior femoral cutaneous nerve	S1, 2, 3
Perforating cutaneous nerve	S2, 3
Pudendal nerve	S2, 3, 4
Pelvic splanchnic nerves	S2, 3, 4
Perineal branch of fourth sacral nerve	S4

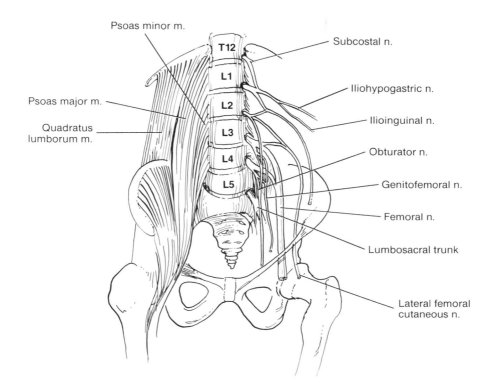

Psoas minor m.

Subcostal n.

T12

L1

Iliohypogastric n.

Psoas major m.

L2

Ilioinguinal n.

Quadratus
lumborum m.

L3

L4

Obturator n.

L5

Genitofemoral n.

Femoral n.

Lumbosacral trunk

Lateral femoral
cutaneous n.

Pelvis (Fig. 32)

The greater sciatic foramen is formed by the greater sciatic notch and the sacrospinous ligament. The lesser sciatic notch and sacrotuberous ligament form the lesser sciatic foramen. All neurovascular structures of the posterior thigh exit through the greater sciatic foramen. Thus the piriformis and all neurovascular structures to the gluteal region and posterior thigh exit through the greater sciatic foramen. The lesser sciatic notch contains the obturator internus muscle, pudendal nerve (principal nerve of the perineum), and internal pudendal vessels. These neurovascular structures will course back into the pelvis. The motor branches of the sacral plexus are as follows:

Superior gluteal nerve: Innervates gluteus medius, gluteus minimus, and tensor fascia lata

Inferior gluteal nerve: Innervates gluteus maximus

"Nerve" to inferior gemellus and quadratus femoris

"Nerve" to obturator internus and superior gemellus

"Nerve" to piriformis

The relationship of the neurovascular structures to the piriformis is essential. The neurovascular structures can be grouped by their position above or below the piriformis.

Above the Piriformis	Below the Piriformis
Superior gluteal artery	Inferior gluteal nerve and artery
Superior gluteal nerve	Pudendal nerve
	Interval pudendal artery
	Nerve to obturator internus
	Sciatic nerve
	Nerve to quadratus femoris
	Posterior femoral cutaneous nerve

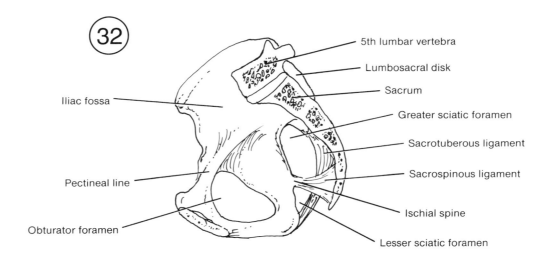

Fig. 32 — labels: 5th lumbar vertebra, Lumbosacral disk, Sacrum, Greater sciatic foramen, Sacrotuberous ligament, Sacrospinous ligament, Ischial spine, Lesser sciatic foramen, Iliac fossa, Pectineal line, Obturator foramen

Muscle attachments (Fig. 33)

The gluteus maximus originates from the posterior gluteal line, sacrum, and sacro-tuberous ligament. The gluteus medius originates between the anterior and posterior gluteal lines; the minimus originates between the anterior and inferior gluteal lines. The hamstrings are composed of the semitendinosus, biceps femoris, semimembranosus, and the ischial portion of the adductor magnus.*

*Classically, semitendinosus, biceps femoris, and semimembranosus make up the hamstring musculature.

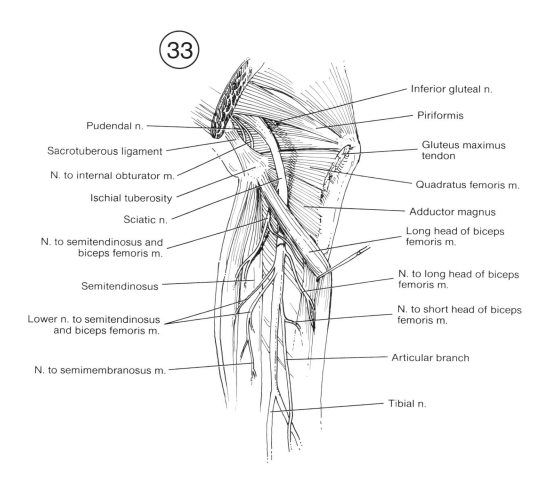

Hamstring Musculature (Fig. 34)

	Origin	Innervation
Semitendinosus	Ischium	Tibial portion of sciatic nerve
Biceps femoris		
Long	Ischium	Tibial portion of sciatic nerve
Short	Femur	Peroneal portion of sciatic nerve
Semimembranosus	Ischium	Tibial portion of sciatic nerve
Adductor magnus*	Ischium	Tibial portion of sciatic nerve

*Classically, semitendinosus, biceps femoris, and semimembranosus make up the hamstring musculature.

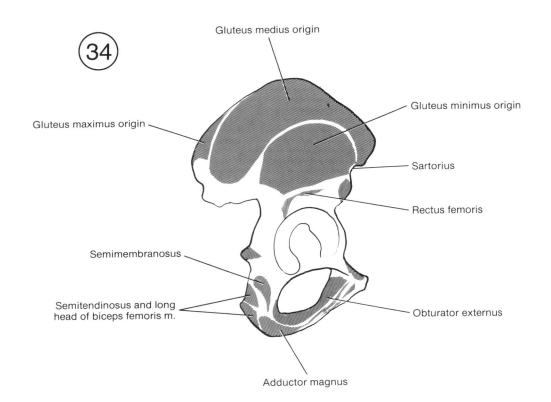

The short external rotators can be seen clearly in Fig. 33. These muscles include the piriformis, superior gemellus, obturator internus, inferior gemellus, and quadratus femoris. The lower border of the quadratus femoris has a plexus of vessels named the "cruciate anastomosis." This collection of vessels is composed of the descending branch of the inferior gluteal artery, the transverse branches of the lateral and medial circumflex femoral arteries, and the first perforating artery.

Anterior superior iliac spine: Origin of sartorius muscle and inguinal ligament

Anterior inferior iliac spine: Origin of direct or straight head of rectus

Posterior superior iliac spine: Sacrotuberous ligament, posterior sacroiliac ligament, multifidus muscle

Posterior inferior iliac spine: Below is the greater sciatic notch (Figs. 35 and 36)

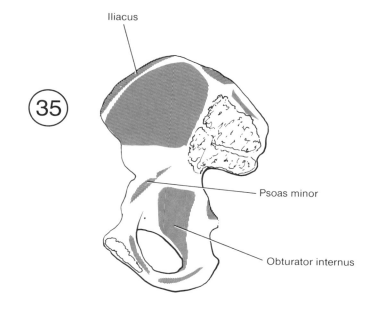

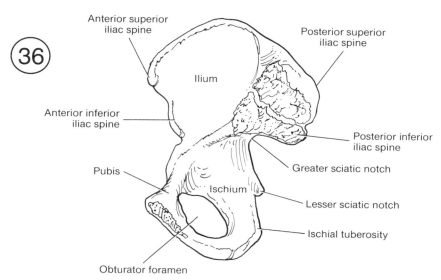

Medial Thigh

The obturator nerve is the principal preaxial (L2 to L4) nerve of the lumbar plexus. It descends along the medial border of the psoas and initially lies on the obturator internus, then travels with the obturator artery and vein through the obturator foramen into the obturator canal of the thigh. The obturator nerve divides into anterior and posterior branches. The anterior branch travels between the adductor longus and the adductor brevis, supplying the "LBG" (adductor *l*ongus, adductor *b*revis, and *g*racilis) and occasionally the pectineus muscle (pectineus usually supplied by the femoral nerve). This anterior division provides cutaneous sensation distally coursing between the gracilis and adductor longus. The posterior division of the obturator nerve travels between the adductor brevis and adductor magnus, supplying the adductor magnus and obturator externus. The posterior division sends an articular branch through the posterior oblique ligament to supply the posterior knee joint.

NOTE: The sensory branches of the obturator nerve are responsible for hip pain that is referred to the knee. Also note that the artery of the ligamentum teres of the hip joint is the terminal branch of the posterior division of the obturator artery.

Surgical Exposures
Hip

The five approaches to the hip are the medial (Ludloff), anterior (Smith-Peterson), anterolateral (Watson-Jones), direct lateral (Hardinge), and posterior (Moore, "Southern," Thomas).

The medial approach to the hip joint has superficial and deep layers. Superficially, dissection should be in the adductor longus/gracilis interval. Deep to this layer, the interval is between the adductor brevis and adductor magnus. It is in the deep layer that you must look for the medial femoral circumflex artery, which is at risk to injury as it travels along the psoas (Fig. 37).

The anterior approach (or "Smith-Pete") also has two planes of dissection. Superficially, between the sartorius and tensor fascia lata, you must look for the lateral femoral cutaneous nerve (Fig. 38). In the deep layer between the gluteus medius and rectus femoris (direct head originates from the anterior inferior iliac spine; reflected head originates from the anterior hip capsule), you must look for the ascending branch of the lateral femoral circumflex artery.

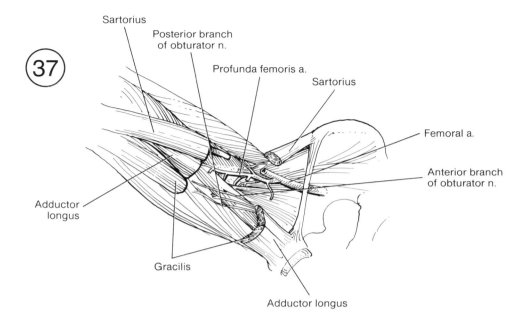

Sartorius

Posterior branch
of obturator n.

Profunda femoris a.

Sartorius

Femoral a.

Anterior branch
of obturator n.

Adductor
longus

Gracilis

Adductor longus

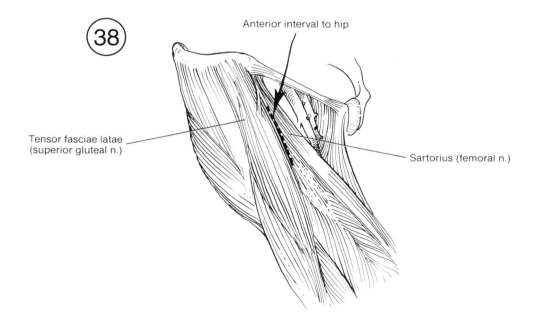

Anterior interval to hip

Tensor fasciae latae
(superior gluteal n.)

Sartorius (femoral n.)

The anterolateral approach (and the direct lateral approach) to the hip requires some type of release of the abductor mechanism. The anterolateral approach utilizes the interval between the tensor fascia lata and gluteus medius with release of the abductor mechanism or trochanteric osteotomy (Fig. 39). Proximal extension between the tensor fascia lata and gluteus medius carries some risk of injury to the superior gluteal nerve. The direct lateral approach requires splitting of the gluteus medius along its fibers with partial release (and eventual repair with closure) of the anterior tendinous insertion of the gluteus medius. Inadequate or poor healing of this repair can result in abductor weakness and a Trendelenburg gait.

The posterior approach to the hip requires release of the short external rotators and care to protect the sciatic nerve. Repair of these muscles should be performed at closure, although this has been infrequent in the past (Figs. 40 and 41).

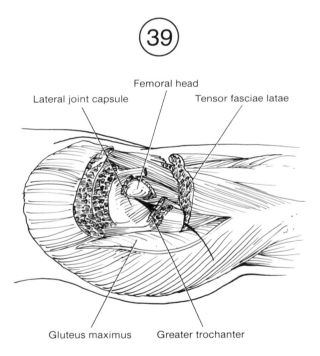

Femoral head

Lateral joint capsule

Tensor fasciae latae

Gluteus maximus

Greater trochanter

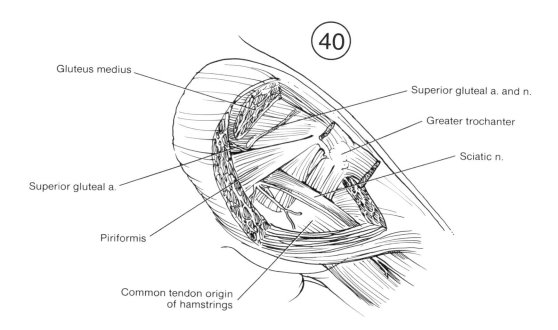

Gluteus medius

Superior gluteal a. and n.

Greater trochanter

Sciatic n.

Superior gluteal a.

Piriformis

Common tendon origin
of hamstrings

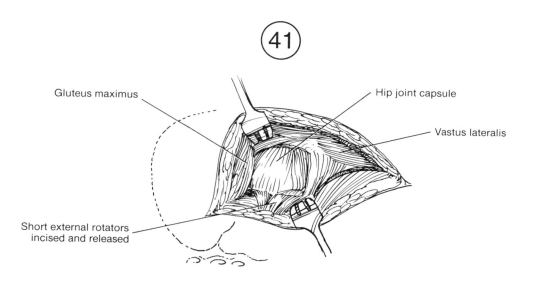

Gluteus maximus

Hip joint capsule

Vastus lateralis

Short external rotators
incised and released

Pelvis

Exposure of the symphysis is performed by means of Pfannenstiel's transverse incision. Sacroiliac exposure is made longitudinally (and posteriorly) 2 cm lateral to the posterior superior iliac spine. Reflection of the piriformis through the greater sciatic notch allows anterior palpation to assess the fracture. Exposure of the iliac bone is made with an incision parallel to the crest. Useful acetabular approaches include the posterior (outlined previously) or Kocher-Langenbeck, the ilioinguinal for exposure of the anterior column, and the extended iliofemoral (curvilinear or triradiate skin incision) for exposure of both columns. The posterior/extended femoral approach and occasionally the posterior approach require osteotomy of the femoral trochanter, and care should be taken to protect the superior gluteal artery. With the ilioinguinal approach (hernia incision), access to the anterior column can be obtained (Fig. 42).

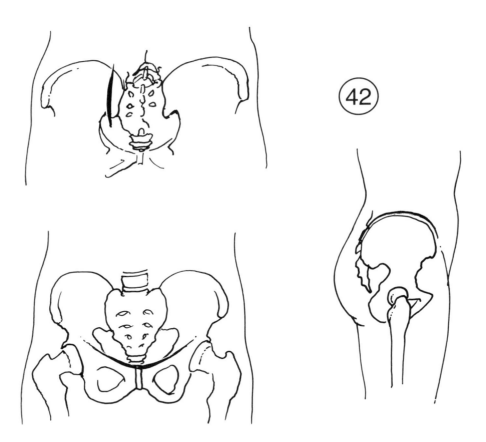

Knee

Knee ligament function has been studied at length over the past decade; however, the anatomy has been accurately defined since the 1970s (Figs. 43 and 44). Most open approaches to the knee require a longitudinal or curvilinear (hockey stick) incision over pathology such as that for tibial plateau fractures. The two approaches gaining a resurgence of popularity for arthroscopic meniscal repairs are the posteromedial and posterolateral exposures to the knee. The posteromedial approach requires a skin incision

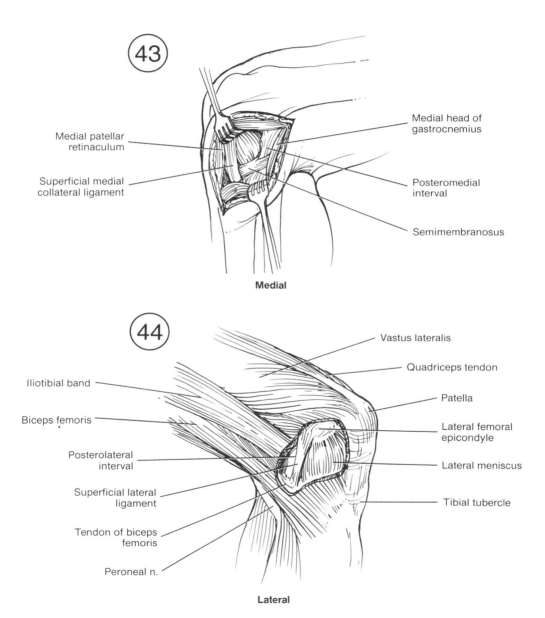

43

Medial patellar retinaculum

Superficial medial collateral ligament

Medial head of gastrocnemius

Posteromedial interval

Semimembranosus

Medial

44

Iliotibial band

Biceps femoris

Posterolateral interval

Superficial lateral ligament

Tendon of biceps femoris

Peroneal n.

Vastus lateralis

Quadriceps tendon

Patella

Lateral femoral epicondyle

Lateral meniscus

Tibial tubercle

Lateral

at the joint line (longitudinal) behind the medial collateral ligament. The fascia is incised between the sartorius and vastus medialis obliquus; thereafter the semimembranous tendon is located and its femoral insertion released. This allows access to the medial gastrocnemius head and placement of a retractor (i.e., Henning type) over the semimembranous tendon and anterior to the gastrocnemius tendon. Posterolateral exposure consists of a vertical skin incision posterior to the fibular collateral ligament using a fascial incision between the iliotibial band and biceps femoris; posterior and medial dissection isolates the lateral gastrocnemius tendon to which a retractor is easily placed anteriorly. The peroneal nerve is at risk as it courses around the lateral gastrocnemius head.

The knee capsule is divided into thirds. Medially, the posterior third capsular ligament is also referred to as the posterior oblique ligament. Laterally, the posterior third capsular ligament thickens and is referred to as the "arcuate ligament." Lastly, the arcuate complex is made up of the lateral collateral ligament (fibular collateral ligament), popliteus tendon, and the arcuate ligament.

Surgical exposures

Approach to the tibial shift is most commonly performed for bone grafting (Fig. 45). The Harmon approach uses an anterior plane of the peroneals, fibula, interosseous membrane, and tibia with the posterior plane comprising the gastrocnemius-soleus complex and the deep posterior compartment contents.

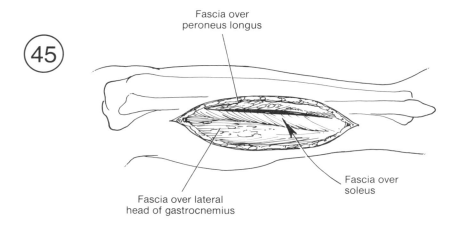

Fascia over
peroneus longus

(45)

Fascia over
soleus

Fascia over lateral
head of gastrocnemius

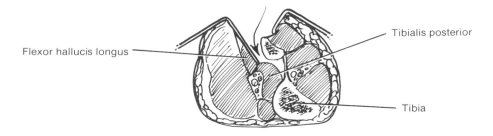

Flexor hallucis longus

Tibialis posterior

Tibia

Four-compartment fasciotomy of the leg uses two incisions. Medially, the skin incision is placed 2 cm posterior to the tibia and is used to release the superficial and deep posterior compartments. Laterally, the incision is placed 2 cm anterior to the fibula and is used to release the anterior and lateral compartments of the leg.

Foot and Ankle

The anatomy of the talus and calcaneus will be dealt with extensively. The anatomy of the foot and neurovascular structures will also be reviewed. Approaches to the ankle will be discussed last.

The ankle joint is of a mortise and tenon construction. The deltoid ligament is made of superficial and deep (intra-articular, runs transversely) fibers. The lateral ligaments are made up of the anterior talofibular ligament (ATFL), calcaneofibular ligament (CFL), and posterior talofibular ligament (PTFL).

ATFL   Fibula to neck of talus
CFL   Fibula to calcaneus
PTFL   Fibula to lateral tubercle of the posterior process of talus

The ligaments of the syndesmosis include the interosseous membrane (IOM), interosseous ligament (distal extension of IOM), anteroinferior tibiofibular ligament (AITFL), posteroinferior tibiofibular ligament (PITFL), and inferior transverse ligament (ITL) (distal extension of PITFL). See Figs. 46 and 47.

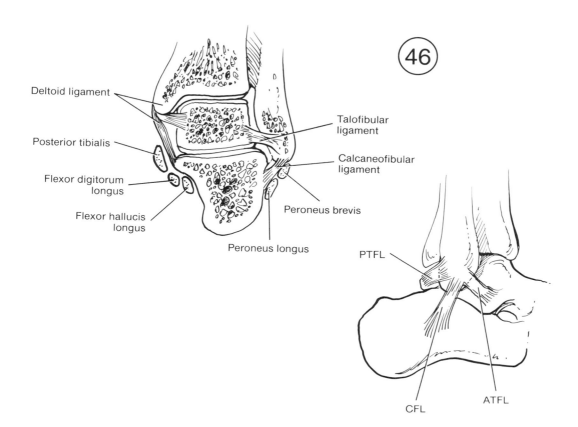

Deltoid ligament

Posterior tibialis

Flexor digitorum
longus

Flexor hallucis
longus

Peroneus longus

Talofibular
ligament

Calcaneofibular
ligament

Peroneus brevis

(46)

PTFL

CFL

ATFL

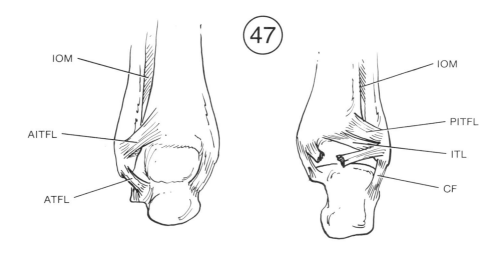

The talus is covered by cartilage over approximately 60% of its surface. No muscles originate or insert on the talus. The lateral process articulates with the lateral malleolus and is the insertion site of the talocalcaneal ligament. The posterior process of the talus is made up of the medial and lateral tubercles. These two tubercles are separated by a groove for the flexor hallucis longus tendon. The lateral tubercle is the most posterior of the two and is the insertion site of the posterior talofibular ligament. The posterior deltoid inserts on the medial tubercle (Figs. 48 and 49).

The posterior tibialis tendon inserts onto the navicular and medial cuneiform bones. The anterior tibialis tendon inserts onto the first tarsometatarsal joint capsule, medial cuneiform, and base of the first metatarsal.

The calcaneus is the strongest and largest bone of the foot; it is shaped like a "pistol grip" and should be conceptualized holding the calcaneus with the thumb sliding under the sustentaculum tali medially. Held as such, the three facets are easily described. Most posterior is the talar (posterior) facet, which has a convex articular surface. Anterior to this facet is the calcaneal sulcus, which leads into the sustentaculum tali. This calcaneal sulcus is positioned under the talar sulcus (containing the interosseus ligament) and laterally becomes the sinus tarsi. Following distal to this sulcus is the middle and anterior talar articular surface (the facet on the calcaneus is named after the bone with which it articulates—namely, "talar"). Thus the calcaneus can be grouped into anterior (anterior and middle facets) and posterior (posterior facet) compartments, divided by the interosseous ligament (Fig. 50).

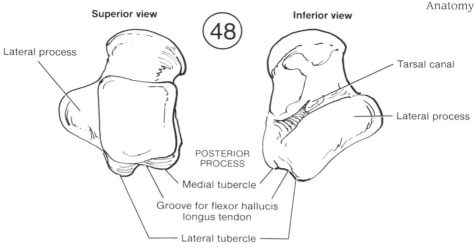

Superior view (48) Inferior view

Lateral process

Tarsal canal

Lateral process

POSTERIOR PROCESS

Medial tubercle

Groove for flexor hallucis longus tendon

Lateral tubercle

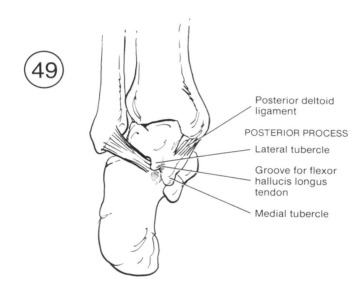

(49)

Posterior deltoid ligament

POSTERIOR PROCESS

Lateral tubercle

Groove for flexor hallucis longus tendon

Medial tubercle

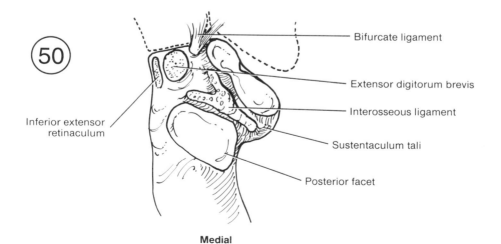

(50)

Bifurcate ligament

Extensor digitorum brevis

Interosseous ligament

Inferior extensor retinaculum

Sustentaculum tali

Posterior facet

Medial

Talocalcaneonavicular joint

This complex is formed by the talus, navicular bone, spring ligament (plantar calcaneonavicular ligament), bifurcate ligament, and anterior and middle calcaneal articular facets. The spring ligament spans from the sustentaculum tali to the navicular bone and functions as a sling or floor (Fig. 51). The wall of the talocalcaneonavicular joint is formed by the Y or bifurcate ligament. The transverse tarsal joints are made up of the calcaneocuboid and talonavicular joints. The transverse tarsal joint is unlocked with the subtalar joint positioned in eversion.

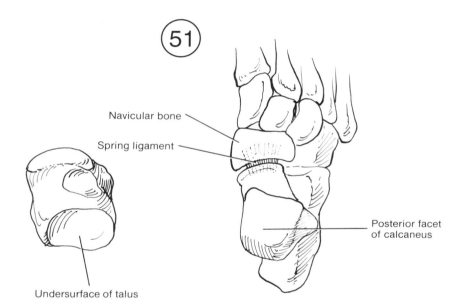

51

Navicular bone

Spring ligament

Posterior facet of calcaneus

Undersurface of talus

Ligaments

The three principal ligaments of the arch of the foot are the spring, plantar calcaneocuboid, and long plantar ligaments. The long plantar ligament stretches from the calcaneal tuberosity to the cuboid and bases of the third, fourth, and fifth metatarsals (Figs. 52 and 53). The bifurcate (Y) ligament stretches from the calcaneus to the cuboid and navicular bones dorsally (Fig. 53).

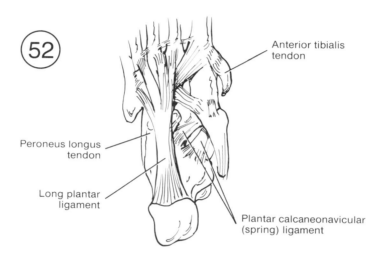

52

Anterior tibialis
tendon

Peroneus longus
tendon

Long plantar
ligament

Plantar calcaneonavicular
(spring) ligament

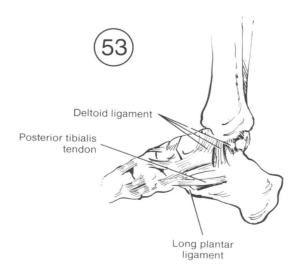

53

Deltoid ligament

Posterior tibialis
tendon

Long plantar
ligament

Intrinsic muscles

The plantar fascia originates from the medial tubercle of the calcaneus and inserts into the proximal phalanges of each toe. The short flexors of the foot insert into the middle phalanges.

The intrinsic muscles of the foot consist of four layers. The neurovascular bundles travel between the first and second layers. The two nerves of the plantar aspect are the medial plantar nerve (MPN) and lateral plantar nerve (LPN). These nerves are analogous to the median and ulnar nerves of the hand, respectively. The LPN enters the foot under the abductor hallucis between the quadratus plantaris and flexor digitorum brevis; thereafter it splits into the superficial and deep branches (superficial carrying motor branches and common digital nerves). The MPN enters under the abductor hallucis forming the motor branches and the common digital nerves. The motor innervation of the MPN is abductor hallucis, first lumbrical, flexor hallucis brevis, and flexor digitorum brevis. The four layers are outlined below and illustrated in Figs. 54 through 57. Lumbricales are situated medially on long flexors.

Another description of plantar foot anatomy is based on compartments (with special reference to fasciotomy, Mubarak and Hargens):

Medial compartment: Abductor hallucis, flexor hallucis brevis

Lateral compartment: Flexor and abductor digiti minimi

Central compartment: Adductor hallucis, quadratus plantae, flexor digitorum brevis, and tendons of the flexor digitorum longus and flexor hallucis longus

Interosseous compartment: Interossei of foot and the plantar arterial arches and digital nerves

Intrinsic Muscles of the Foot

Layer	No.	Muscle/Tendon	Motor Innervation
1	3	Abductor digiti minimi	LPN
		Flexor digitorum brevis	MPN
		Abductor hallucis	MPN
2	2 + 2	Quadratus plantae	LPN
		Flexor digitorum longus	Tibial nerve
		Flexor hallucis longus	Tibial nerve
		Lumbricales	
		Second through fourth	LPN
		First	MPN
3	3	Flexor digiti minimi	LPN
		Adductor hallucis	LPN
		Flexor hallucis brevis	MPN
4	2 + 2	Dorsal interossei	LPN
		Plantar interossei	LPN
		Posterior tibialis	Tibial nerve
		Peroneus longus	Superficial peroneal nerve

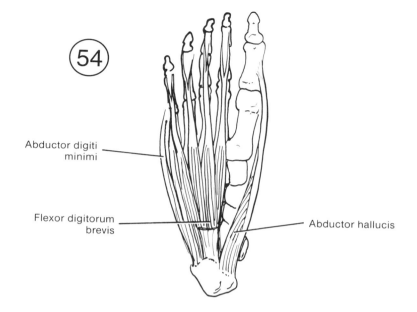

54

Abductor digiti
minimi

Flexor digitorum
brevis

Abductor hallucis

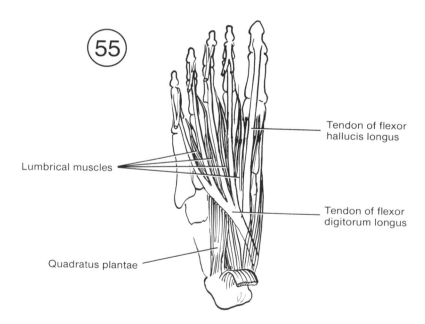

55

Lumbrical muscles

Quadratus plantae

Tendon of flexor
hallucis longus

Tendon of flexor
digitorum longus

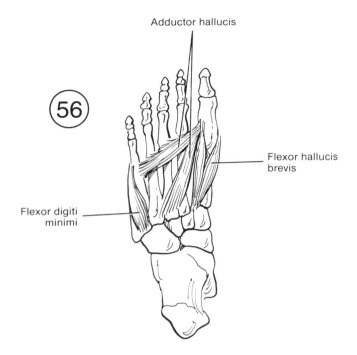

Adductor hallucis

Flexor hallucis brevis

Flexor digiti minimi

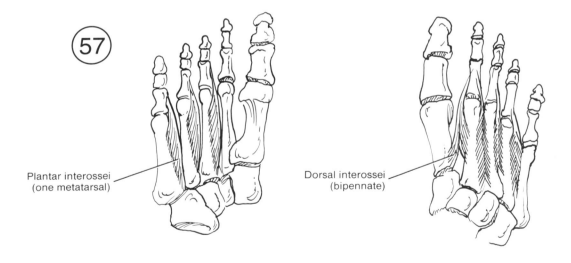

Plantar interossei (one metatarsal)

Dorsal interossei (bipennate)

Surgical exposures

The anterior approach to the ankle requires knowledge of the anterior neurovascular bundle. The anterior tibial artery and nerve lie between the extensor digitorum longus and anterior tibialis. The neurovascular bundle is crossed by both the extensor hallucis longus and brevis distally in the foot. The approach to the ankle uses a retinacular incision, mobilizes the neurovascular bundle, and retracts it and the extensor hallucis longus medially. The extensor digitorum longus is retracted laterally. Alternatively, the joint can be entered medial to the anterior tibialis (Fig. 58).

Medial and posteromedial approaches are related to their position to the medial malleolus. The posteromedial approach requires great care to protect the posterior tibial artery and nerve; the plane is between the flexor hallucis longus and the Achilles tendon. The posterolateral approach to the ankle is the distal extension of the Harmon bone graft approach discussed previously (using the plane between the flexor hallucis longus and peroneus longus). The short saphenous vein and nerve are at risk as they course posterior to the lateral malleolus. Remember that the peroneus brevis is anterior to the longus and hugs the fibula.

The anterolateral approach to the ankle is lateral to the extensor digitorum longus and peroneus tertius. The lateral approach to the posterior talocalcaneal joint requires incision of the peroneal tendon sheaths and mobilization of the peroneal tendons to expose the underlying talocalcaneal joint.

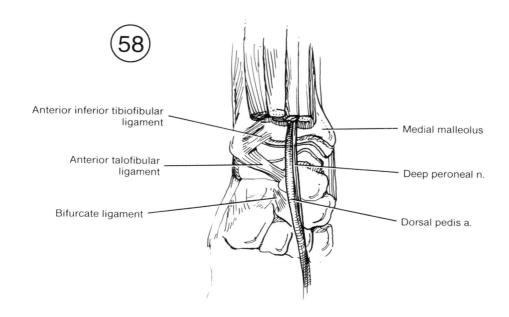

(58)

Anterior inferior tibiofibular ligament

Anterior talofibular ligament

Bifurcate ligament

Medial malleolus

Deep peroneal n.

Dorsal pedis a.

2

FRACTURE
CLASSIFICATION

Hand

1. Flexor digitorum profundus avulsion
   Type I: Tendon retracts into palm
   Type II: Tendon retracts to proximal interphalangeal joint
   Type III: Large bony avulsion, retracting to A4 pulley
2. Dorsal metacarpophalangeal dislocations
   Simple: Subluxation
   Complex: Irreducible (skin dimpling)
3. Scaphoid (by location)
   Tuberosity
   Distal third
   Wrist
   Proximal third
   Distal osteochondral fracture

Forearm

1. Frykman classification of Colles' fractures

	Distal Ulnar Styloid Fracture	
Fracture	Absent	Present
Extra-articular	I	II
Intra-articular and radiocarpal involvement	III	IV
Intra-articular distal radioulnar joint involvement	V	VI
Intra-articular with radiocarpal and distal radioulnar joint involvement	VII	VIII

2. Monteggia's fracture
   Type I (60%): Anterior dislocation of radial head, ulna fracture at any level
   Type II (15%): Posterior or posterolateral dislocation of radial head
   Type III (20%): Lateral or anterolateral dislocation of radial head
   Type IV (5%): Anterior dislocation of radial head; fracture of proximal third of radius (fracture of both bones of the forearm)

Upper Arm

1. Supracondylar humerus fracture
   a. Extension: Distal fragment posterior
      Type I: Nondisplaced
      Type II: Partially displaced or angulated
      Type III: Completely displaced
   b. Flexion: Distal fragment anterior

2. Intercondylar fracture of the distal humerus (Riseborough and Radin)
   Type I: Undisplaced fracture
   Type II: Separation of capitellum and trochlea without rotation
   Type III: Separation and rotation
   Type IV: Separation, rotation, and comminution
3. Humeral condyle fracture
   a. Lateral condyle (Fig. 59)
      Milch type I: Lateral trochlear ridge remains intact (Salter-Harris type IV fracture)
      Milch type II: Lateral trochlear ridge is part of fractured lateral condyle (Salter-Harris type II fracture)
   b. Medial condyle (Fig. 60)
      Milch type I: Lateral trochlear ridge remains intact (providing stability) (Salter-Harris type IV fracture)
      Milch type II: Lateral trochlear ridge is part of fractured medial condyle (Salter-Harris type II fracture)

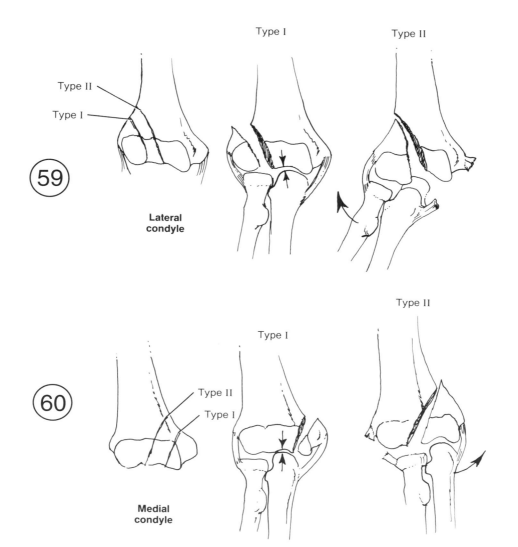

c. Stage of displacement
    (1) Jakob et al., 1975
        Stage I: Relatively undisplaced, articular surface is intact
        Stage II: Complete fracture
        Stage III: Complete displacement, rotated
    (2) Badelon et al., 1988
        Stage I: Fracture undisplaced and seen on only one x-ray view
        Stage II: Fracture seen on two x-ray views and displacement is less than 2 mm
        Stage III: Displacement is greater than 2 mm on both x-ray views
        Stage IV: Complete separation of fragments
4. Capitellar fracture
  Type I (Hahn-Steinthal type): May involve trochlea, larger bone fragment
  Type II (Kocher-Lorenze type): Minimal subchondral bone, "shell" fracture
5. Radial head fracture
  Type I: Nondisplaced
  Type II: Marginal fracture with displacement
  Type III: Comminuted whole-head fracture
  Type IV: Any of the above with elbow dislocation

(61)

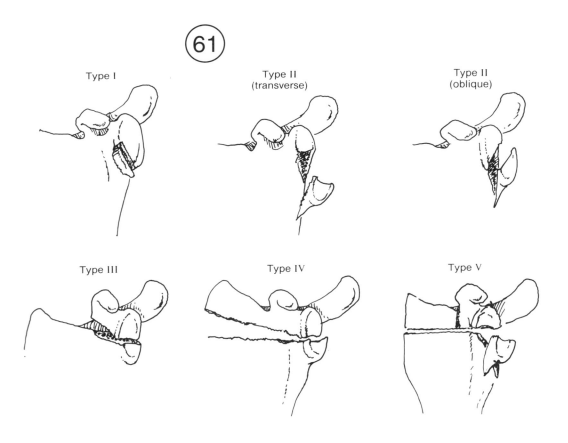

Type I   Type II (transverse)   Type II (oblique)

Type III   Type IV   Type V

6. Proximal humerus

Neer's classification (anatomic segments—anatomic neck, surgical neck, greater tuberosity, lesser tuberosity, fracture dislocation, and head-splitting)

One-part: Nondisplaced, any number of fracture lines

Two-part: Displacement of 1 cm or 45-degree angulation of two anatomic segments

Three-part: Three anatomic segments, each separated 1 cm or angulated 45 degrees

Four-part: Four anatomic segments separated or angulated

7. Glenoid fracture (Ideberg) (Fig. 61)

Type I: Anterior avulsion fragment

Type II: Complete fracture through glenoid leaving a free inferior glenoid fragment

Type III: Fracture through upper third of glenoid

Type IV: Horizontal fracture extending through to axillary border of scapula

Type V: Combination of types II and IV

Girdle

1. Clavicle fracture

   a. Distal third

      Type I: Minimal displacement

      Type II: Displacement secondary to fracture medial to coracoclavicular ligaments
      - Conoid and trapezoid ligaments attached
      - Conoid torn, trapezoid attached

      Type III: Articular surface fractures

      Type IV: Periosteal ligament interface intact (children)

      Type V: Comminution, ligaments avulsed

   b. Proximal third

      Type I: Minimal displacement

      Type II: Significant displacement

      Type III: Intra-articular

      Type IV: Epiphyseal separation

      Type V: Comminuted

2. Scapula (Zdravkovic and Damholt)

   Type I: Fracture of the body

   Type II: Fracture of the apophyses

   Type III: Fracture of superior lateral angle (including glenoid neck)

3. Acromioclavicular joint disorders

   Type I: Ligaments and acromioclavicular joint intact (sprain)

   Type II: Subluxations of acromioclavicular joint
   - Coracoclavicular ligaments intact (vertical stability)
   - Acromioclavicular capsule torn (horizontal instability)

   Type III: Complete dislocation of acromioclavicular joint superiorly

   Type IV: Posterior dislocation of distal end of clavicle

   Type V: More severe version of type IV; distal clavicle stripped of attachments and lies subcutaneously at neck

   Type VI: Inferior dislocation of distal clavicle

Spine

1. Fracture of the dens (Fig. 62)
   Type I: Oblique fracture through upper part of dens
   Type II: Fracture through isthmus of odontoid
   Type III: Fracture extends into body of axis
2. Traumatic spondylolisthesis of the axis (hangman's fracture) (Fig. 63)
   Type I: No angulation
   Type II: Angulation greater than 10 degrees and displacement greater than 3 mm
   Type IIA: Type II with widening of L2-3 interspace posteriorly (angulation only)
   Type III: Dislocation of C2-3 facets with severe angulation
3. Thoracolumbar fracture
   Compression
   Burst
   Flexion distraction (including Chance fracture)
   Fracture-dislocation

Pelvis

1. Pelvic ring disruption (Tile)
   Type A (stable)
      A1: Fracture of pelvis not involving ring
      A2: Minimally displaced fracture of the ring, stable
   Type B (rotationally unstable, vertically stable)
      B1: Open book
      B2: Lateral compression—ipsilateral
      B3: Lateral compression—contralateral
   Type C (rotationally and vertically unstable)
      C1: Rotationally and vertically unstable
      C2: Bilateral
      C3: Associated with an acetabular fracture

Pelvis (Young)

1. Lateral compression: Transverse fracture of pubic rami
   Type I: Sacral compression on impact side
   Type II: Iliac wing fracture on impact side
   Type III: Lateral compression I or II on side of impact contralateral open book (anteroposterior compression)
2. Anteroposterior compression: Symphyseal diastasis and/or longitudinal rami fracture
   Type I: Slight widening of pubic symphysis; intact sacroiliac ligaments
   Type II: Widened sacroiliac joint anteriorly; disrupted anterior sacroiliac ligaments; intact posterior sacroiliac ligaments
   Type III: Complete sacroiliac joint disruption; disrupted sacroiliac ligaments (posterior and anterior)

3. Vertical shear: Symphyseal diastasis and vertical displacement through sacroiliac joint, ileal fracture, or sacral fracture
4. Combination: Combination of patterns, most commonly lateral compression/vertical shear

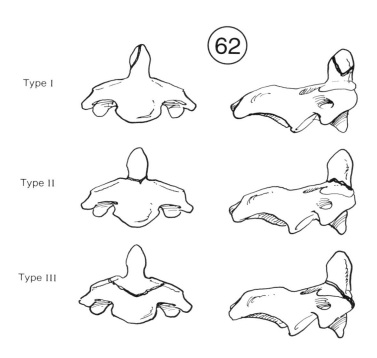

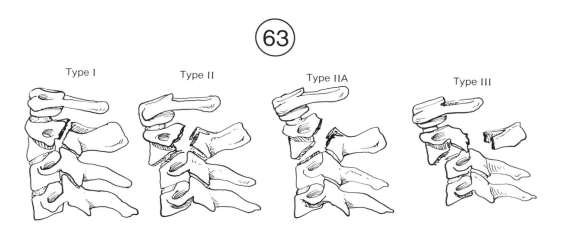

Acetabulum

1. Fracture types (A-O)
   Type A: One column fractured, the other intact
      A1: Posterior wall
      A2: Posterior column
      A3: Anterior wall and/or anterior column
   Type B: Transverse types with portions of roof attached to intact ilium
      B1: Transverse and posterior wall
      B2: T types
      B3: Anterior type with posterior hemitransverse
   Type C: Both columns are fractured and all articular segments, including the roof, are detached from the remaining segment of the intact ilium
      C1: Anterior column fracture extends into iliac crest
      C2: Anterior column fracture extends to anterior border of the ilium
      C3: Fracture enters the sacroiliac joint
2. Fracture types (Tile)
   a. Undisplaced
   b. Displaced
      Type I: Posterior types ± posterior dislocation
      • Posterior column
      • Posterior wall
         Associated with posterior column
         Associated with transverse fracture
      Type II: Anterior types ± anterior dislocation
      • Anterior column
      • Anterior wall
      • Associated anterior and transverse fracture
      Type III: Anterior types ± central dislocation
      • Pure transverse
      • T fracture
      • Associated transverse and acetabular wall fractures
      • Double-column fracture

Hip

1. Femoral neck fracture (Garden)
   Type I: Incomplete or impacted neck fracture
   Type II: Complete fracture without displacement
   Type III: Complete fracture with partial displacement
   Type IV: Complete fracture with total displacement of the fracture fragments
2. Intertrochanteric femoral fracture (Kyle et al.)
   Type I: Nondisplaced, stable
   Type II: Displaced, minimally comminuted, stable
   Type III: Large posteromedial comminution, unstable
   Type IV: Intertrochanteric fracture with subtrochanteric component

3. Subtrochanteric fracture (Seinsheimer)
   Type I: Nondisplaced or displaced less than 2 mm
   Type II: Two-part fracture
   Type IIA: Two-part transverse
   Type IIB: Two-part spiral, lesser trochanter
   Type IIC: Two-part spiral, lesser trochanter attached to distal fragment
   Type III: Three-part fracture
   Type IIIA: Three-part spiral fracture, lesser trochanter part of third fragment
   Type IIIB: Three-part spiral fracture, third part a butterfly fragment
   Type IV: Comminuted fracture with four or more fragments
   Type V: Subtrochanteric-intertrochanteric fracture

Hip Dislocations

1. Anterior dislocations
   Type I: Superior dislocations
   Type IA: No associated fracture
   Type IB: Associated femoral head and/or neck fracture
   Type IC: Associated acetabular fracture
   Type II: Inferior dislocations
   Type IIA: No associated fracture
   Type IIB: Associated femoral head and/or neck fracture
   Type IIC: Associated acetabular fracture
2. Posterior dislocations (Thompson and Epstein)
   Type I: With or without minor fracture
   Type II: Large single fracture of posterior acetabular rim
   Type III: Comminution of the acetabular rim
   Type IV: With fracture of acetabular floor
   Type V: With fracture of femoral head
3. Subclassification of type V (Pipkin)
   Type I: Posterior dislocation of the hip with fracture of femoral head caudad to fovea centralis
   Type II: Fracture of femoral head cephalad to fovea centralis
   Type III: Type I or II associated with a femoral neck fracture
   Type IV: Type I, II, or III associated with fracture of the acetabulum
4. Femoral shaft fracture (Winquist, Hansen, and Clawson)
   Type I: Minimal or no comminution
   Type II: Comminution greater than type I, but 50% of the circumference of the cortices of the major fracture fragments is intact
   Type III: Fifty percent to 100% of the circumferences of the two major fracture fragments are comminuted
   Type IV: All cortical contact is lost

Knee

1. Tibial plateau (A-O) (Fig. 64)
   Type I: Wedge
   Type II: Depression
   Type III: Wedge and depression
   Type IV: Y and T fractures or comminuted fractures of both condyles
2. Fracture dislocation of the knee (Moore)
   Type I: Split
   Type II: Entire condyle
   Type III: Rim avulsion
   Type IV: Rim compression, contralateral collateral tear
   Type V: Four-part fracture

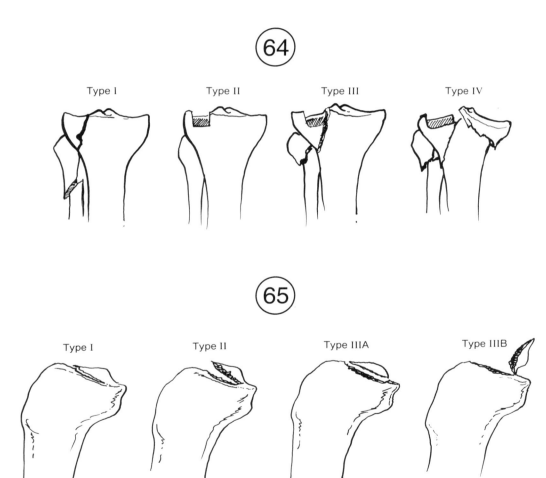

(64)

Type I   Type II   Type III   Type IV

(65)

Type I   Type II   Type IIIA   Type IIIB

3. Tibial spine (eminence) fracture (Meyers and McKeever) (Fig. 65)
   Type I: Anterior edge of eminence is slightly elevated
   Type II: Greater elevation of anterior eminence
   Type IIIA: Entire eminence is fractured out of tibial bed
   Type IIIB: Complete eminence fracture with rotation
4. Collateral ligament injury
   Grade I or first degree: Microscopic tear, intact ligament function
   Grade II or second degree: Partial tear (macroscopic); partial ligament functional
   compromise, but endpoint present
   Grade III or third degree: Complete tear, ligament function lost
5. Knee dislocation: Determined by position of tibia on femur
   Anterior
   Posterior
   Medial
   Lateral
   Rotatory

Ankle Fractures

Lauge-Hansen (classification with injury stages)
   Supination-adduction
      Stage 1: Transverse fracture of fibula below joint line
      Stage 2: Vertical fracture of medial malleolus
   Supination-eversion: Eversion = external rotation
      Stage 1: Disruption of anterior tibiofibular ligament
      Stage 2: Spiral oblique fracture of distal fibula
      Stage 3: Disruption of posterior tibiofibular ligament or fracture of posterior
      malleolus
      Stage 4: Fracture of the medial malleolus or deltoid ligament tear
   Pronation-abduction
      Stage 1: Transverse fracture of medial malleolus or deltoid ligament tear
      Stage 2: Rupture of syndesmosis
      Stage 3: Short, horizontal, oblique fibular fracture above joint line
   Pronation-eversion
      Stage 1: Transverse fracture of medial malleolus or deltoid ligament
      Stage 2: Disruption of anterior tibiofibular ligament
      Stage 3: Short oblique fracture of fibula above joint line
      Stage 4: Rupture of posterior tibiofibular ligament or tibial fracture
   Pronation-dorsiflexion
      Stage 1: Fracture of medial malleolus
      Stage 2: Fracture of anterior margin of tibia
      Stage 3: Supramalleolar fracture of fibula
      Stage 4: Transverse fracture of posterior tibial surface

Danis-Weber

Weber A: Fracture of fibula below tibial plafond level (Lauge-Hansen "supination-adduction")

Weber B: Spiral fibular fracture at level of tibial plafond (Lauge-Hansen "supination-eversion")

Weber C: Fracture of fibula above the syndesmosis (Lauge-Hansen "pronation-eversion" or "pronation-abduction")

Talar neck fracture (Hawkins)

Type I: Nondisplaced vertical fracture of talar neck

Type II: Displaced fracture of the talar neck with subluxation or dislocation of the subtalar joint

Type III: Displaced fracture of the talar neck with dislocation of the body from the subtalar and ankle joints

Lisfranc's tarsometatarsal joint

Homolateral: All five metatarsals displaced in the same direction

Isolated: One or two metatarsals displaced from the others

Divergent: Displacement of the metatarsals in both the sagittal and coronal planes

3

METABOLIC BONE DISEASE

This complex topic requires extensive study, and the following discussion is only a foundation for understanding the processes and a mental structure for further reading. In addition, it is meant to be a practical discussion enabling you to answer questions based on patient presentations and the varying laboratory values (Joseph Moskal, M.D., personal communication, 1990).

There are three general headings into which the disease processes can be divided. Although initially it is common practice to refer to calcium values in metabolic bone disease, it is best to categorize by *phosphate levels*. By considering the level of the patient's phosphorus and then using calcium values, you will be able to differentiate, diagnose, and decide on treatment.

Before proceeding it is important to define commonly used (and mystifying) terms. For most discussions rickets and osteomalacia are synonymous but are used for different age groups—childhood vs. adulthood, respectively. Renal osteodystrophy and secondary hyperparathyroidism also are interchangeable for most basic discussions. Renal osteodystrophy has three components and can present a very confusing clinical picture. The components are (1) secondary hyperparathyroidism, (2) abnormal mineralization of bone with aluminum, and (3) osteomalacia (phosphate binders in the gut chelate calcium also). Nonetheless, most questions concerning renal osteodystrophy involve the component of secondary hyperparathyroidism. Primary hyperparathyroidism has various causes (80% adenoma, 4% adenocarcinoma, 15% hyperplasia), but metabolically it is one process. Lastly, osteomalacia can be broken down into vitamin D deficient, vitamin D dependent, and vitamin D resistant rickets (children) as differentiated by laboratory values.

The first two groups are osteoporosis and Paget's disease. Both are collagen disorders, not disorders of mineralization; both processes have normal phosphate and calcium levels. In fact, laboratory tests for osteoporosis will demonstrate all normal values (Ca, Pi, alk phos, ESR, and PTH). However, because of their increased bone metabolism, patients with Paget's disease will have elevated alkaline phosphatase and urinary hydroxyproline. Thus:

Phosphorus Normal
Calcium Normal

Osteoporosis	*Paget's Disease*
P: Normal	P: Normal
Ca: Normal	Ca: Normal
Alk phos: Normal	Alk phos: ↑
PTH: Normal	Urinary hydroxyproline: ↑

Continuing with the discussion, there are two processes that can result in an elevated level of phosphorus (either renal failure or increased metabolism secondary to carcinoma). Renal osteodystrophy (secondary hyperparathyroidism) has a low normal calcium level. The remaining studies will be elevated, including alkaline phosphatase, PTH, and BUN and creatinine levels. With reference to multiple myeloma or carcinomas, there is an elevated calcium level. In multiple myeloma there will be an **M** spike (IgG) on serum protein electrophoresis. Thus the second grouping, elevated phosphorus, is as follows:

Phosphorus Elevated

Renal Osteodystrophy
P: ↑
Ca: ↓
Alk phos: ↑
PTH: ↑
BUN/creatinine: ↑

Multiple Myeloma
P: ↑
Ca: ↑

Hypoparathyroidism, pseudohypoparathyroidism, and pseudopseudohypoparathyroidism usually completely confuse the situation, but again the category is elevated phosphorus and differentiation is on the basis of given facts. Hypoparathyroidism has a decreased calcium level and is associated with basal ganglia calcification. Pseudohypoparathyroidism (Seabright bantam syndrome, sex-linked dominant) has a decreased calcium level also, but there will be the additional clinical information of short metacarpals and metatarsals of the first, fourth, and fifth digits. Pseudopseudohypoparathyroidism has a normal calcium level (see below).

Phosphorus Elevated

Hypoparathyroidism
P: ↑
Ca: ↓
Basal ganglia calcification

Pseudohypoparathyroidism
P: ↑
Ca: ↓
Short metacarpals and metatarsals 1, 4, and 5

Pseudopseudohypoparathyroidism
P: ↑
Ca: Normal

Last is the discussion of hypophosphatemia. You must differentiate between vitamin D deficient and vitamin D resistant rickets. In vitamin D deficient rickets, the calcium level is low or normal. In vitamin D resistant rickets, the calcium level is classically normal (and the process is sex-linked dominant). Remember, in vitamin D resistant rickets, the abnormality is in phosphate loss ("phosphate diabetes," a defect in phosphate absorption) and calcium values are usually not affected.

Phosphorus Decreased

Osteomalacia/Rickets

VITAMIN D DEFICIENT
P: ↓
Ca: ↓
Alk phos: ↑
PTH: ↑

VITAMIN D DEPENDENT
P: ↓
Ca: ↓
Alk phos: ↑
PTH: ↑
(Defect of 1-OH-lase)

VITAMIN D RESISTANT
P: ↓
Ca: Normal
Alk phos: ↑
PTH: ↑

Primary hypoparathyroidism also has a decreased phosphorus but is easily differentiated from rickets or vitamin D resistant rickets because it is associated with an elevated calcium level.

Phosphorus Decreased

Primary Hyperparathyroidism

P: ↓
Ca: ↑
Alk phos: ↑
PTH: ↑

Primary and secondary hyperparathyroidism have the same histologic appearance; they are differentiated by laboratory findings.

Using the previous discussions and material, a helpful chart may be developed:

Phosphorus Normal Calcium Normal	**Phosphorus Elevated**	**Phosphorus Decreased**
Osteoporosis P: Normal Ca: Normal Alk phos: Normal PTH: Normal	*Renal Osteodystrophy* P: ↑ Ca: ↓ Alk phos: ↑ PTH: ↑ Bun/creatinine: ↑	*Osteomalacia/Rickets* VITAMIN D DEFICIENT P: ↓ Ca: ↓ Alk phos: ↑ PTH: ↑
Paget's Disease P: Normal Ca: Normal Alk phos: ↑ Urinary hydroxypro- line: ↑	*Multiple Myeloma* P: ↑ Ca: ↑ *Hypoparathyroidism* P: ↑ Ca: ↓ Basal ganglia calcification	VITAMIN D DEPENDENT P: ↓ Ca: ↓ Alk phos: ↑ PTH: ↑ (Defect of 1-OH-lase)
	Pseudohypoparathyroidism P: ↑ Ca: ↓ Short metacarpals and metatarsals 1, 4, and 5	VITAMIN D RESISTANT P: ↓ Ca: Normal Alk phos: ↑ PTH: ↑
	Pseudopseudohypopara- thyroidism P: ↑ Ca: Normal	*Primary Hyperparathyroidism* P: ↓ Ca: ↑ Alk phos: ↑ PTH: ↑

Normal values for laboratory studies are as follows: Ca, 8.5 to 10.5; P, 3.0 to 4.5; and alkaline phosphatase, 20 to 90 IU.

Treatment depends on the diagnosis and is usually covered on examinations (depending on what is current).

Osteoporosis
   Ca: 1500 mg/day
   Vitamin D: 400 U/day
   Estrogen: Within 3 years of menopause
   Fluoride: Initial results show increased bone mass but not strength (more brittle) and currently not recommended
   Cyclical diphosphonates

Paget's disease
   Calcitonin for 6 months (follow alkaline phosphatase and hydroxyproline)
   Diphosphonates
   Mithramycin for paraplegia

Osteomalacia
   Vitamin D deficient: Vitamin D and calcium
   Vitamin D resistant: 50,000 units of vitamin D and calcium

Multiple myeloma: Chemotherapy

Primary hyperparathyroidism: Parathyroidectomy

Renal osteodystrophy
   Dialysis, reduce phosphate (phosphate binders)
   Calcium supplements

BIBLIOGRAPHY

Abbott LC, Carpenter WF. Surgical approaches to the knee joint. J Bone Joint Surg 27:277-310, 1945.

Badelon O, Bensahel H, Mazda K, et al. Lateral humeral condylar fractures in children: A report of 47 cases. J Pediatr Orthop 8:31-34, 1988.

Bado JL. The Monteggia lesion. Clin Orthop 50:71-86, 1967.

Frykman G. Fracture of the distal radius including sequelae—shoulder-hand-finger syndrome, disturbance in the distal radio-ulnar joint, and impairment of nerve function: A clinical and experimental study. Acta Orthop Scand 108(Suppl):1-155, 1967.

Grant JCB. Grant's Atlas of Anatomy. Baltimore: Williams & Wilkins, 1972.

Hardinge K. The direct lateral approach to the hip. J Bone Joint Surg 64B:17-19, 1982.

Hawkins LG. Fractures of the neck of the talus. J Bone Joint Surg 52A:991-1002, 1970.

Henry AK. Extensile Exposure, 2nd ed. Baltimore: Williams & Wilkins, 1970.

Henry AK. Extensile Exposure, 3rd ed. Edinburgh: Churchill Livingstone, 1972.

Hoppenfeld S, deBoer P. Surgical Exposures in Orthopaedics: The Anatomic Approach. Philadelphia: JB Lippincott, 1984.

Hughston JC. A surgical approach to the medial and posterior ligaments of the knee. J Bone Joint Surg 55A:923-940, 1973.

Ideberg R. Fractures of the scapula involving the glenoid fossa. In Bateman JE, Welsh RP, eds. Surgery of the Shoulder. Toronto: BC Decker, 1984, pp 63-66.

Jakob R, Fowles JV, Rang M, Kassab MT. Observations concerning fractures of the lateral humeral condyle in children. J Bone Joint Surg 57B:430-436, 1975.

Kyle RF. Intertrochanteric fractures. In Chapman MW, ed. Operative Orthopaedics. Philadelphia: JB Lipppincott, 1988, pp 353-359.

Lauge-Hansen N. Fractures of the ankle. II. Combined experimental-surgical and experimental-roentgenologic investigations. Arch Surg 60:957-985, 1950.

Meyers MH, McKeever FM. Fractures of the intercondylar eminence of the tibia. J Bone Joint Surg 52A:1677-1684, 1970.

Milch H. Fractures and fracture dislocations of the humeral condyles. J Trauma 4:592-607, 1964.

Moore AT. The self-locking metal hip prosthesis. J Bone Joint Surg 39A:811-827, 1957.

Moore TM. Fracture-dislocation of the knee. Clin Orthop 156:129-140, 1981.

Muller ME, Allgoner M, Schnieder R, Willenger H. Manual of Internal Fixation Techniques Recommended by the A-O Group, 2nd ed. New York: Springer-Verlag, 1970.

Neer CS II. Prosthetic replacement of the humeral head: Indications and operative technique. Surg Clin North Am 43:1581-1597, 1963.

Pipkin G. Treatment of grade IV fracture-dislocation of the hip. J Bone Joint Surg 39:1027-1042, 1197, 1957.

Rockwood CA Jr, Green DP, eds. Fractures in Adults, 2nd ed. Philadelphia: JB Lippincott, 1984.

Rockwood CA Jr, Green DP, Bucholz RW, eds. Fractures in Adults, 3rd ed. Philadelphia: JB Lippincott, 1991.

Rockwood CA Jr, Wilkins KE, King RE, eds. Fractures in Children. Philadelphia: JB Lippincott, 1984.

Rockwood CA Jr, Wilkins KE, King RE, eds. Fractures in Children, 2nd ed. Philadelphia: JB Lippincott, 1991.

Seinsheimer F. Subtrochanteric fractures of the femur. J Bone Joint Surg 60A:300-306, 1978.

Smith-Petersen MN. Approach to and exposure of the hip joint for mold arthroplasty. J Bone Joint Surg 31A:40-46, 1949.

Taleisnik J, Kelly PJ. The extraosseous and interosseous blood supply of the scaphoid bone. J Bone Joint Surg 48A:1125-1137, 1966.

Thompson JE. Anatomical methods of approach in operating on the long bones of the extremities. Ann Surg 68:309-329, 1918.

Thompson VP, Epstein HC. Traumatic dislocation of the hip. J Bone Joint Surg 33A:746-778, 1951.

Tile M. Fractures of the Pelvis and Acetabulum. Baltimore: Williams & Wilkins, 1984.

Warren LF, Marshall JL. The supporting structure and layers on the medial side of the knee. J Bone Joint Surg 61A:56-62, 1979.

Winquist R, Hansen S, Clawson K. Closed intramedullary nailing of femoral fractures. J Bone Joint Surg 66A:529-539, 1984.

Young JWR, Burgess AR. Radiologic Management of Pelvic Ring Fractures: Systematic Radiographic Diagnosis. Baltimore: Urban & Schwarzenberg, 1987.

Zdravkovic D, Damholt VV. Comminuted and severely displaced fractures of the scapula. Acta Orthop Scand 45:60-65, 1974.

CREDITS

Figs. 6, 8, 9, 11, 12, 14 through 17, 19 through 21, 23, 24, 26, 27, 29, and 37 through 41 were redrawn from Hoppenfeld S, deBoer P. Surgical Exposures in Orthopaedics: The Anatomic Approach. Philadelphia: JB Lippincott, 1984.

Fig. 42 was redrawn from Orthopaedic Knowledge Update, Home Study Syllabus. Chicago: American Academy of Orthopaedic Surgeons, 1984.

Figs. 46 through 50, 54 through 57, 59 through 61, and 63 through 65 were redrawn from Rockwood CA Jr, Green DP, eds. Fractures in Adults, 2nd ed. Philadelphia: JB Lippincott, 1984.

INDEX